The Motivator Meal Plan!

Before you begin to read this guide, I would like to congratulate you on being one of those individuals who is ready to make a positive change. By following the principles and guidelines that are outlined here and remaining consistent, you are going to take your physique to a whole new level and create the body you have always wanted.

So here we have it. You're determined to lose that excess body fat? Or really increase your muscle mass for those "Gains". You have your gym membership, new sports kit and trainers; you may have even booked a Personal Trainer for that one hour session? Or you have been training frequently, understand how to exercise correctly and you are forever running on that treadmill? Whichever situation best describes you; there may be a little something missing? Now, that little something; seems so small. So small most of the time that it's completely overlooked and as long as you get your daily dose of exercise you think it's ok to leave this small thing out? What is the SMALL THING? That small thing is what you are putting into your mouth the other 23 hours per day that you are not at the local gym! That small thing is your Nutrition! Don't worry; I have experienced overlooking my nutrition for many years in the past. But I'm here today to tell you that the seemingly "small thing" that you haven't been taking care of is actually 80% of your overall result and the way in which you look! Not so small now? I didn't think so. Let me tell you a fact that it is actually 80% Nutrition accompanied by 20% exercise and physical activity that makes all of the difference. Before fully understanding the importance of nutrition; I stood tall at 6ft 3" but weighed in excess of 21stones and NO this was not made up of pure lean muscle; rather the opposite. My daily routine would consist of skipping breakfast, picking up a slice of pastry from my local bakery on my way to work, starving myself for the next 5 hours, having fast food in the afternoon and then arriving back home so late that I would literally throw myself into bed with the crisps and chocolates I could find in the cupboard, before falling asleep and repeating the process the following morning. Oh, I forgot to mention that on the weekends or if I managed to finish a work a little early during the week I would spend 2 hours a time in the gym, but my nutrition outside of this would still be the same. I know, it's no wonder that I ended up with such excessive amounts of body fat, visceral fat and a real lack of energy!

So what has changed? Currently I am in the best physical condition and health I have ever witnessed in my whole life. I have more energy each day to complete day to day tasks, I no longer have those afternoon naps due to feeling so tired, my lean muscle mass is the highest it has ever been and I am totally confident with my personal appearance and physique. And the best news is, I am here to share with you exactly how I have achieved this in such a relatively short space of time. Now, I am not a nutritionist and have never claimed to be; this book is based purely on what has worked for me and is based upon my opinion and first-hand experience. Before making any significant changes to your nutrition I would suggest consulting your doctor, certainly if you have any underlying medical issues.

Let me tell you a little secret. When I lived day to day eating as and when I pleased and snacking on whatever it was that came into my vision; not once at any moment in time that I can remember did anybody at all pull me aside and say "Kurt, I don't think you should be eating that. It contains next to no nutrition and certainly isn't going to help you to reduce your body fat or increase your lean muscle." Of course this doesn't mean that anybody was to blame for my terrible eating habits. But from experience one thing that I learnt was that I was massively missing the education and the simple steps to follow in order to change my eating habits. My response at the time would have been "OK, no problem. But what should I be eating instead?" This knowledge is so vital. Vital for anyone who wants to live a healthier and more active lifestyle, improve their physique or increase their energy. And this Is why The Motivator Meal Plan has been designed to not only answer some of these more common questions; but to actually guide you through what can be such a simple and complex subject into a much more simple guide that you can follow.

Don't worry, this is not going to be one of those books/guides based around the field of nutrition that turn into a science lesson and bore you to tears. This is going to be something very different, put forward in a way that you will not have ever seen before.

How frequently are you eating?

Ok, so you have arrived in the Sahara desert. You haven't consumed food in hours and you really are not sure when you are going to eat next. Your body suddenly goes into a "starvation" type of mode and says to itself "The next time I eat, I am going to store this as fat just in case I don't eat again for a very long time". So finally you reach food and as you begin to eat and over indulge because you are so hungry; your body stores a little more than usual as fat (almost like the storage of a camels hump). Oh, but I forgot to mention; you're not really in the middle of the Sahara Desert, you have just left too much of a gap between meals! And this is how your body reacts! This is the importance of eating regularly throughout the day to avoid putting your body into this position. Have you ever met somebody who says "I can't believe this, I hardly ever eat and I just keep gaining weight?" Well now you have the answer, "Stop making your body believe it's in the middle of a desert and needs to store fat." So what is the solution? Eat regularly during your waking hours (eat every 2-3 hours) this is far more effective that only eating one meal throughout the day just like so many people do! Remember, whatever we do not use we lose! If we do not give our metabolisms something to do frequently; they are going to slow right down. And then when we do need them most... They are no longer working as efficiently as we would like.

Are you drinking enough water?

I told you! Never before have you heard nutrition put in this way. "Sahara Desert" he says! But here is another little story to help you with the topic of hydration. Tony was standing in the kitchen one day and he was about to receive a great shock whilst washing up! (Not quite the shock his wife would have received, by finding out that he is actually doing the washing up for once) So, everything was moving along as always, he took the dishes and washed them one by one, followed by the glasses and cups and then finally he looked over to the one object that he had been putting off to clean for the last ten minutes. The Oven Tray! He took the greasy oven tray that was covered in meat fats and started to rinse it under the tap! As he was doing so he noticed that the water and the meat fats "Didn't quite mix" it was almost as if one was rejecting the other and causing a gooey substance to form! That is very similar my view of what happens inside of our bodies. You will find that an individual who has excessive amounts of body fat will automatically be less hydrated day to day. Yes this is even if they drink a little more water. This is why it is super important to keep yourself well hydrated with at least 2-3litres of water per day (of course depending on the size of the individual) but also reducing your body fat so that the body can operate without this "rejection process" happening. I definitely suggest keeping yourself hydrated as dehydration is also another factor that can contribute to further gaining of body fat.

If you now understand the philosophy and reason why it is important to stay hydrated. But are struggling with the thought of drinking that amount of water throughout the day, I would like to let you into a little secret I use with so many of my clients to help them drink at least 2 litres of water per day. I would like you to take a two litre bottle and with a permanent marker draw a number of lines directly across the bottle which will be your markers. You can either simply remember the times that each marker symbolises or add timings to your bottle too with the permanent marker. This simple challenge has allowed many of my clients who initially struggled to see how they could drink even 2 litres of water per day to now drink this with ease. This little experiment breaks the larger end goal of two litres into smaller 250 – 300ml sections that are super easy to drink every couple of hours when having your snack/meal! Try it! (The image below is an example of an individual who wakes up at 8am and has created their bottle based on 2 Litres over the next 12 hours. Think about just how easy that would be? But, surprisingly most people do not even drink anywhere near 2 litres of water per day)

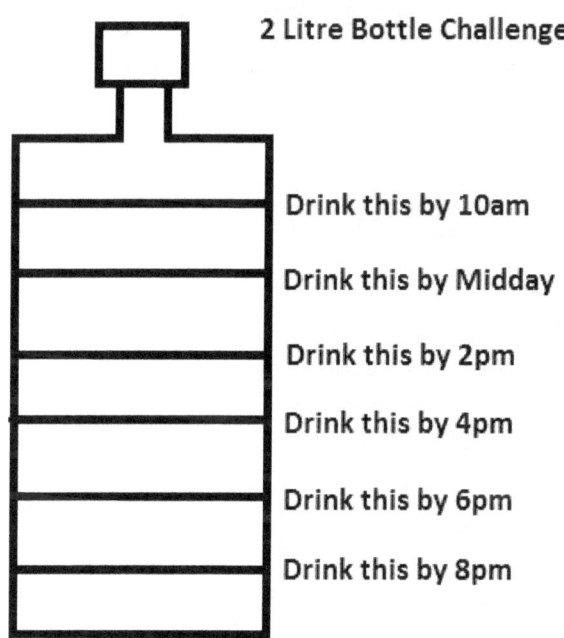

2 Litre Bottle Challenge

Drink this by 10am

Drink this by Midday

Drink this by 2pm

Drink this by 4pm

Drink this by 6pm

Drink this by 8pm

How important is breakfast?

Next, I would like to introduce you to another friend of mine. He usually goes to sleep around 10pm in the evening and wakes up around 6am in the morning. He wakes up and feels ok but little does he know that during his night's sleep, his body has been taking part in the 3 R's Resting, Rejuvenating and Rebuilding from any bodily stresses on the previous day. This process requires many nutrients, meaning that when he wakes up there is now an important 30 minute window to replace all of the nutrients he has lost before continuing with his day. However, he decides to skip breakfast because he is in a hurry for work. By this time his blood sugars are very low because he has not eaten the right nutrition or in fact anything at all. When he arrives at work he is now so hungry and low in energy that he reaches for the sweetest thing he could find and starts to eat a chocolate bar. Now his sugars levels are sky high and have reached their limits meaning that his body is now going to release something called insulin which will help to stabilise his blood sugars! This does not assist as this is also a factor of gaining weight and body fat. It's now mid-afternoon and his blood sugars are now once again very low so it's time to reach for another excessive carbohydrate or sugar snack to attempt to "fight his cravings"... Guess what happens next? You guessed it! The body fights against the sugars once again and this cycle continues throughout the day! This puts him on a whirlwind of suddenly going from being full to being hungry throughout the day, his energy levels are low and over a longer period of time he would have gained a significant amount of body fat. Does this sound familiar? Well it's a very simple fix, but not as simple as you may have been programmed to believe. Many people believe wholeheartedly that by simply having a bowl of cereal (high carbohydrates) or a piece of toast and tea (again high in carbohydrates) that they can avoid the situation that has been described above. I'm sorry to rain on your parade a little, but in fact starting your day with simply having excessive amount of carbs just triggers the spikes in your blood sugars a little quicker and then you are off on pretty much the same rollercoaster once again! So what is the solution? The solution is to ensure you have a balanced 40% Protein 30% Carbohydrate and 30% fats breakfast accompanied by a tall glass of water each morning. The balanced breakfast can either be made up of whole food sources or a meal replacement shake/bar. In the mornings I personally opt for a shake as it is very convenient and allows me to avoid both of the situations above. Feel free to contact me directly at kurtisshinner@live.co.uk for more information regarding the meal replacement supplements I personally use.

What's so important about Protein, Carbohydrates and Fats?

It's now time to touch on the basis of Proteins, Carbohydrates and fats. All of which are of course very important in our diet but do we know why?

Proteins – The Kurt Motivator definition of protein is that proteins are the building blocks of muscle and are used by pretty much every single cell in our bodies as they promote both their repair and growth. Most people massively neglect protein and in my experience of working with clients I can confidently say that in excess of 80% of people who I come into contact with simply do not know how much protein they should have per day? OK, to nip this in the bud; there are many ways to calculate your protein target but the method I choose is to first of all find out your lean muscle mass. Your lean muscle mass can be calculated on an electronic set of scales, many pharmacies now have these so this is easy enough to find. Once you know your lean muscle mass, convert it into pounds (lbs) and that's your number! Your body requires that many grams of protein per day!

Now let's take the example of myself. My muscle mass is now approximately 12 stone 4lbs. Now to convert this to lbs. 12 x 14 and then add the 4lbs. This gives 172lbs meaning that I have 172lbs of muscle, but also meaning that my body requires 172 grams of protein per day to stay nice and lean. If we look back to my previous lifestyle or pastry and fast food throughout the day; on a good day I would have been consuming 30-40 grams of protein maximum and therefore would lead to me not only losing muscle mass quickly but also slowing my metabolism as a result! And that's how simple it is. Consume nice clean proteins to meet your protein target and believe me you are 90% on your way to having your dream body!

Our diets as a whole an individual meals should consist of approximately 40% carbohydrates, 30% proteins and 30% fats. This is what we would call a healthy balanced meal and would most certainly put you on the correct track. However, if you are wanting to reduce your body fat and get super lean. When physically looking at your dinner plate I would like you to remember the numbers 50%

Protein, 25% Vegetables and 25% (a fist full) of typical carbohydrates (We do know that vegetable is also a carbohydrate right? This is why I mention typical carbohydrate, we will touch on these in just a moment). Or, if you really want to get Super Dooper Lean and reduce your body fat then what Kurt Motivator does is 50% Protein and 50% Vegetables. This is because, so frequently individuals will totally overlook protein and totally line their plates with heavy carbohydrates first.

The Motivator Lean Meal Example:

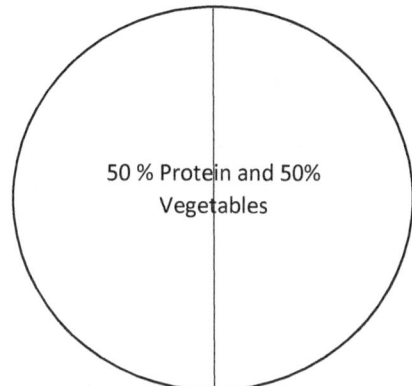

50 % Protein and 50% Vegetables

Remember, this is where we slightly change our philosophy. From the typical regime of lining our plates with carbohydrates to now adding our proteins first (exact amounts based on our protein targets)

To help you along here is a list of the top protein sources that I use daily:

Fish

Quinoa

Hemp Seeds

Chia Seeds

Pumpkin Seeds

Lentils

Chicken

Low Fat Cottage Cheese

Greek Yoghurt

Egg Whites

Almond Nuts

Brazil Nuts

Green Peas – Although not expected; a cup of green peas contains the same amount of protein as a glass of milk.

Beef – I generally only eat red meat in moderation due to its acidity. I do not exceed any more than one serving per week.

How to find the Grams of protein in food?

To many people the answer to this question may be obvious, although before I gained a better understanding of nutrition I had no idea at all of where to find the nutritional value of a food source. Firstly, the protein value can be found on the rear of most packaged meats but make sure you check the total weight of the portion you will be eating and compare that the protein value per 100g which is usually stated on the packaging. Of course if you have purchased your lean meats or poultry from a butchers then the easiest method would be to search the protein per 100g online prior to your purchase. If you decide to opt for a vegetable source of protein; once again you can generally find the exact amount of protein per serving at the rear of the packaging.

Carbohydrates

Let's talk a little bit about carbohydrates. In fact I hear so often that carbohydrates are simply "not good" or somebody has decided to "cut carbs" which I think is very silly. Yes I can understand the philosophy of reducing the amount of carbohydrates that you are eating so that you are not storing any unused carbs as fat. However, carbohydrates play a massive roll in energy and providing the body with the energy it needs to carry out specific tasks. Carbohydrates also play a huge factor in the functioning of the brain and I believe that totally "cutting" out any major macro nutrient is not massively sustainable. When looking at the Motivator Meal Plan you can see that 25% of the whole plate is what we would call typical carbohydrates. The word typical is used here to describe what many people would automatically class as a "carb":

White Bread/Brown Bread

White Pasta/Brown Pasta

White Rice/Brown Rice

I would personally suggest from this day forward, if you are going to eat any of the above "typical carbohydrates" then stick to "Brown" or "Wholemeal".

However, the following foods are also excellent sources of carbohydrate and are generally overlooked or placed into a different category altogether:

Fruit

Vegetables

Dairy Products (Notice that dairy products can appear both in the Protein and Carbohydrate category as they contain reasonable amounts of both macros just ensure that you are reading the packaging and determining the amount of Protein and Carbohydrates per serving before consuming)

Fats

We sometimes alienate the word "fats" and automatically think that any foods that contain fat is simply not good for us. Now that is true to an extent with particular types of fat, however there are also some very health fats which are essential for the way our body's function. Let me give you an example. In the summer of 2013 I decided to take my body fat down to a whole new level of ripped! If that is what you would like to call it. I followed the Motivator Nutrition Plan Perfectly having 5-6 balanced meals per day, reached my protein target daily, followed the water challenge and my 20% training was also spot on. I managed to maintain this physique throughout autumn and then into the beginning of the winter. One day I was in an office working at my previous job and remember sitting and talking to a number of colleagues (don't tell the boss we were talking). After about 10-15 minutes of sitting in this office I started to feel a little cold. So I asked my colleagues "guys, is there a window open in here? It feels really cold". "No" everyone replied "It's actually quite warm in here Kurt". This totally baffled me but I didn't mention anything for a while, zipped my jacket up and decided to carry on with my work. Over the next 30 minutes I felt really cold and decided to ask again "are you sure there isn't a window open anywhere in here guys? There seems to be a draft". Once again everyone responded "NO" and continued with their work. I was very confused, my thoughts at the time were "maybe I'm coming down with something?" and then all of a sudden it clicked! My super low levels of body fat that felt great in the summer, was suddenly starting to work against me! It wasn't that there was a window open or a draft, the other guys in the office simply had higher levels of body fat and didn't feel the cold at all. So there you have it, one of the disadvantages of having low body fat in the middle of the winter and an example of why some fats are important too! Don't forget that fats also provide a great source of energy and 1g of fat does provide the equivalent of 9kcal.

A little about the different types of fats:

You would have learnt by now that this guide isn't written from a scientific approach and I don't intend it to be. Its 1 thing knowing the science and another thing applying it, I couldn't even put into words the amount of medical professionals with doctorates and degrees that don't apply the most simple of practices on themselves! Surely, that would be a better example to the community and population? I'm simply the guy who applies the knowledge, I don't just fill myself up with facts to sound intelligent; I take action and I get results for myself and thousands of others around the world! Anyway, back to discussing the different types of fats.

There are basically a couple of different categories of fats called saturated, monounsaturated and polyunsaturated which really depends on their chemical structure (Science over!). But all can be broken down into two key areas BAD fats and GOOD fats. It doesn't take a rocket scientist to understand that in our daily diets we need to avoid those BAD fats and maybe increase the lack of GOOD fats!

Those "Bad Fats":

In my opinion saturated fats fall into the category of BAD fats. It's recommended that males should consume no more than 30g of saturated fats per day and females 20g. However, of course if you want that wonderful physique; you definitely don't need to be hitting the maximum amount each day! Be cautious when consuming any products that contain more than 8g of fat per 100g and definitely if they contain more than 17g of fat per 100g.

A grilled beef burger, chunk of cheddar cheese, butter or any items heavy in pastry with butter are a couple of examples.

Healthier Sources of Fat:

Omega 3 fatty acids are a type of fat that have fantastic benefits for the body. They can assist with joint health, arthritis, stiffness in mobility and even heart and brain health.

They are most prominently found in oily fish such as salmon or mackerel.

Now we are ready to add our 50% Protein, 25% Typical Carbohydrates and 25% Vegetables or 50% Protein and 50% Vegetables to our plate. Here are some of the most effective combinations I use to get a super lean physique.

The Lean Meal Plan 50% Proteins 25% Typical Carbohydrates 25% Vegetables

1 ½ Turkey Breasts (50%) A fist full of brown rice (25%) and Mixed Vegetables (25%)

1 ½ Large Chicken Breasts (50%) A fist full of brown rice (25%) and mixed Vegetables (25%)

1 ½ Pieces of white fish (Average in size – 50%) A fist full of brown rice (25%) and mixed vegetables (25%)

1 full tin of tuna (50%) A fist full of brown rice (25%) and mixed vegetables (25%)

½ Plate of Tofu (50%) A fist full of brow rice (25%) and mixed vegetables (25%)

1 ½ Turkey Breasts (50%) 1 Medium sized sweet Potato (25%) and Mixed Vegetables (25%)

1 ½ Large Chicken Breasts (50%) One Medium Sized Sweet Potato (25%) and mixed Vegetables (25%)

1 ½ Pieces of white fish (Average in size – 50%) One Medium Sized Sweet Potato (25%) and mixed vegetables.

1 full tin of tuna (50%) 3 tbsp One Medium Sized Sweet Potato (25%) and mixed vegetables (25%)

½ Plate of Tofu (50%) One Medium Sized Sweet Potato (25%) and mixed vegetables (25%)

1 ½ Turkey Breasts (50%) 3 tbsp Wholemeal Cous Cous (25%) and Mixed Vegetables (25%)

1 ½ Large Chicken Breasts (50%) 3 tbsp Wholemeal Cous Cous (25%) and mixed Vegetables (25%)

1 ½ Pieces of white fish (Average in size – 50%) 3 tbsp Wholemeal Cous Cous (25%) and mixed vegetables (25%)

1 full tin of tuna (50%) 3 tbsp Wholemeal Cous Cous (25%) and mixed vegetables (25%)

½ Plate of Tofu (50%) 3 tbsp Wholemeal Cous Cous (25%) and mixed vegetables (25%)

½ plate of High Protein Quorn (50%) and Mixed Salad (50%)

1 clean steak fillet (50%) with a Medium Sized Sweet Potato (25%) and mixed salad (25%)

Chicken Wraps – 1 ½ Chicken Breasts (50%) with 1 Wholemeal Wrap (25%) and mixed salad (25%)

Egg White Omelette (3-4 Egg Whites and 1 yolk – 50%) with 1 slice of wholemeal toast (seeded if possible for extra protein – 25%) and a mixed salad (25%)

1 Large Salmon Fillet (50%) a fist full of wholemeal pasta (25%) and mixed vegetables (25%)

Prawns and low fat cottage cheese (1/2 plate – 50%) a fist full of brown rice (25%) and a mixed salad (25%)

Nice and Easy – A mix of tuna and low fat cottage cheese (50%) 1 wholemeal pitta (25%) and a mixed salad (25%)

The Super Lean Meal Plan – 50% Proteins and 50% Vegetables

1 ½ Turkey Breasts (50%) and ½ Plate of mixed vegetables (50%)

1 ½ Large Chicken Breasts (50%) and ½ plate of mixed vegetables (50%)

1 ½ Pieces of white fish (Average in size – 50%) and ½ plate of mixed vegetables (50%)

1 full tin of tuna (50%) and ½ plate of mixed vegetables (50%)

½ Plate of Tofu (50%) and ½ plate of mixed vegetables (50%)

½ Plate of High protein Quorn (50%) and ½ plate of mixed vegetables (50%)

1 ½ Chicken Breasts (50%) and ½ plate of mixed salad (50%)

1 Clean Steak Fillet (50%) with ½ plate of mixed Salad (50%)

Egg White Omelette (3-4 Egg Whites and 1 yolk – 50%) and ½ plate of mixed salad (50%)

1 Large Salmon Fillet (50%) and ½ plate of mixed salad (50%)

Prawns and low fat cottage cheese (1/2 plate – 50%) and a mixed salad (50%)

Nice and Easy – A mix of tuna and low fat cottage cheese (50%) and a mixed salad (50%)

By this time you should have started to better understand the ratios! Give some of these a try!

I recommend some of the following vegetables to build your 25% Mixed Vegetables section of the plate:

Carrots

Broccoli

Spinach

Kale

Asparagus

Cucumber

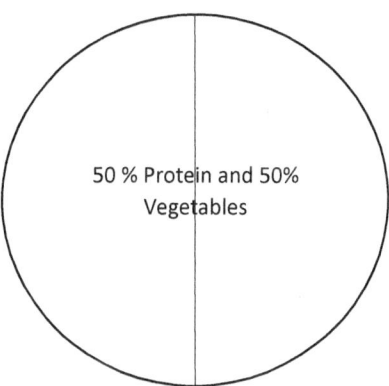

50 % Protein and 50% Vegetables

Beetroot

Tomatoes

Green Peas

Sweetcorn

Onions

Peppers

Brussels sprouts

Avocado (A fantastic source of healthy fats)

Cauliflower

Green Beans

Lettuce

Mushrooms

Radishes

Celery

And of course the list continues! But these are my personal favourites!

Can I have sauces with my meals?

Remember that to calculate the correct amount of calories you will need to consume each day in order to lose/gain weight you will simply need to use an electronic scale to calculate your BMR. Again this is the amount of calories that your body will burn each day at rest. To lose weight/body fat you should take this number and reduce it by 500 (never going below 1000kcal per day) and that will give you your daily allowance of calories. This is the part where I will need you to do a little thinking and be honest with yourself. If you are well within your daily calories after adding your 5-6 meals/snacks per day and taking into consideration your protein target. Then it is absolutely fine to add additional sauces. However, I would like to make clear that many sauces that are readily available contain sugars and sweeteners that may hinder your overall results on the Motivator Meal Plan. So yes, everything in moderation is fine. But I would always opt for the lower calorie/lower fat option if available.

Why do I limit the amount of red meat I consume?

Although red meat does contain a great source of protein along with other beneficial properties such as niacin in a leg of lamb. I do find that red meat is often found with an excessive amounts of fat, which of course isn't great for that perfect physique. However, this reason alone is not the only reason that I limit the amount of red meat I consume after all you can still find a pretty lean piece of steak! The main reason I do not consume too much is really down to the acidity of red meat. Eating too many acid forming foods in your diet can be very detrimental for a number of reasons. In the next section I will go on to discuss the differences between Acid and Alkaline foods, some ideas of where they can be found and also their effects on our body.

Acid vs. Alkaline

Without turning this guide into a science lesson I would briefly like to touch on the difference between acid and alkaline forming foods. The Acidity or Alkalinity of something is measured using the PH Scale, A PH below 7 is classed as acidic and a PH of 7 or above is alkaline. The human blood is generally alkaline and typically eating too many acidic foods, combined with stresses, toxins and a number of other determining factors can cause the blood to become more acidic. When this happens it can decrease the body's natural ability to repair damaged cells, produce energy and can even lead to fatigue and illness. In some more rare cases if the body becomes too acidic it can even lead to more fatal circumstances.

Just to make you aware of what you are putting into your body; here is a list of some common acid forming foods:

Sugar

Corned Beef

Sausage

Lamb

Peanut Butter

Spaghetti

Bread

Flour, Wheat

Kidney Beans

Fizzy Drinks

Eggs

Beef

Artificial Sweeteners

Jelly

Alcohol

Pork

Here is a list of a few alkaline foods to give you a better understanding:

Lettuce

Mushrooms

Cabbage

Sweet Potatoes

Wild Greens

Cucumber

Celery

Apples

Apricots

Blackberries

Dandelion Root

Spices

Herbs

Nuts

Now that you have a better understanding of the PH scale and an Idea of where you can find more acidity and alkalinity in foods, in the next section I would like to take you through some information you may or may not already know about the PH of water.

The PH of Water

Another thing I massively take into consideration is the PH of water, particularly bottled water. When purchasing a bottle of water, something that is very simple and easy to do yet effective; is to look at the back of the bottle for the PH of the water. Remember that anything under a PH of 7 when bottled at source is generally acidic and should be avoided (of course there are a number of other determining factors). What surprises me, is that very often some of the more familiar and popular brands of water have a far lower PH and tend to be more acidic than some of the cheaper brands of bottled water. Remember: Anything lower than the number 7 under the PH section is Acidic and anything higher than the number 7 is alkaline.

A Tip to increase Your Lean Muscle and Weight

So here is a tip that is very rarely mentioned but in fact can almost double the progress you are making currently. When trying to gain lean muscle mass or increase the amount of calories you are consuming, you may sometimes feel that there are simply not enough hours in the day! However, this simple little trick will allow you to go above and beyond your targets and into a new dimension of results. Have you ever thought of setting your alarm clock for intervals throughout the night (whilst sleeping) simply to roll over and grab your protein shake or snack that is next to the bed? How about that for an idea! It is a known fact that so many body builders around the world do this to achieve fantastic results. Let's face it, it only takes a couple of minutes away from your rest (which is equally important) but the gains and advantages could be Huge! When contemplating which food source to have next to your bedside table; again I would personally opt for a protein snack to protect your lean muscle mass throughout the night. I know you are looking forward to this! Finally, a midnight snack that is actually allowed!

The Motivator Daily Guide Example (Stick to the fridge)

I would now like to talk you through a day in the life of my nutrition. Of course the nutritional supplements may vary. This is simply my personal choice of meal replacement supplement due to my research and experience. So here we have an official day in the life of Kurt Motivator.

First of all I ensure that I Eat every 2-3 hours (5 times per day)

Drink 2.5 - 3L (8 glasses) of water per day

Morning (or the time you first wake up)

My plan begins within the first 30 minutes of waking up. It's vital to ensure you are replacing a large percentage of the nutrients lost whilst sleeping; within this period of time.

I begin my day with 2 tablespoons of Formula 1 along with Personalised Protein Powder in 250-450ml semi skimmed/soya milk. This provides me with all of the nutrients required and sets me up perfectly for the day ahead. This full meal replacement shake also provides 25g of clean protein which keeps me aligned with my protein target)

+3 hours later (Now it's time for my snack – typically I choose 2 of the options below and combine them as my protein snack, which provides 20g of protein at this time of the day)

Snack (use the options here as a guide):

- Almond nuts (50g)

- Hazelnuts (50g)

- Cottage cheese

- Peanut butter and Rice Cakes (x 2)

- Diced chicken breast

- 1 tin of tuna

- A Fruit Salad (No Bananas or Raisins - high in sugar)

- Greek Yoghurt (Total Zero/Danio) and Berries

+ 3 hours later

For Lunch I would have 2 tablespoons of Formula 1 along with Personalised Protein Powder in 250-450ml semi skimmed/soya milk. Again this provides an additional 25g of clean protein. I will generally have either ½ tin of tuna or a piece of white fish at this time of the day too. Bringing my Lunch time total in excess of 35g protein.

+3 hours later

And then onto the 2nd Snack of the day (I would now once again choose 2 options from the initial snack menu above or another protein snack typically containing 20g of protein)

Evening Meal (Balanced 50-25-25)

When looking at my dinner plate; I try to use the following ratios:

50% of the plate Protein/Fats (Less Red Meats - If you choose to eat red meat; just once per week)

- Chicken

- Turkey

- Prawns

- Fish

- Beans

25% of the plate Carbohydrates

- Brown Rice

- Brown Pasta

- Wholemeal Cous Cous

- Sweet Potato

Vegetarian:

- Quorn

- Tofu

25% of the plate Vegetables

Vegetables must be colourful! Green alone is not enough. This meal would generally provide me with 30-40g of lean protein along with balanced nutrition and correct portion sizes to build a lean muscular physique. As always, the correct portion and serving size depends on the individual and their protein target. Once you have this information it is simple enough to check the product labelling for the protein per servings and integrate these servings across your 5 meals per day until your target is achieved. At this point in the evening (after my evening meal), all that is remaining is my additional Rebuild Strength Protein shake which I take 30 minutes before heading to sleep. I simply add 5 level scoops of rebuild strength to water and drink!

Ok, so you are probably thinking "he uses products and meal replacements, why is that? First, of all I would like to tell you that not everyone who chooses to follow this nutrition plan is required to use the same products and meal replacements. If your protein target and ratios of 50% Protein 25% Typical Carbohydrates and 25% Vegetables are correct it is possible to simply calculate your protein target for example 150g and divide that by 5. Meaning that if your protein target it 150g you will need to consume 5 meals containing 30g of protein per day in order to achieve your personal protein target. Of course if you do not currently have a meal replacement shake then your breakfast should still be balanced also. 2 poached eggs with salmon (50%), 1 wholemeal toast (25%) and veggies (25%) or a combination containing the above ratios is far better than a typical breakfast cereal.

However, one of the reasons I personally choose to use meal replacement supplementation is because they provide my body with many of the smaller micronutrients that are now depleting in the food sources of today. In order to get the most nutrient dense food sources along with lower caloric intake, meal replacements have most certainly been the most feasible option.

What if I work night shifts or funny work hours?

If you find yourself working throughout the night or waking up very early in the mornings. Simply remember and abide by the 30 minute rule and every 2-3 hour rules. For example, whether you wake up at 6am, 4am, 2am or 4pm in the afternoon it is important that you consume your balanced nutritional meal within 30 minutes of waking up. It's also important that you maintain the consistency of eating every 2-3 hours while you are awake. Of course this where preparation is key so that you do not find yourself reaching for the biscuit tin when you realise that you failed to prepare your snacks or meals in advance.

Meal Prep! When and Why?

As a great teacher once taught us "If you fail to plan, you plan to fail". It's amazing that some people will plan their next night out with more care than they have planned what they are about to put into their body! The term "Meal Prep" really doesn't need to sound that daunting, it doesn't necessarily need to involve the freezing and defrosting of food and the worries of how long each item can be stored! It really doesn't! Let me give you an example of what I do as it might clear up a few of those worries! First of all, on a Saturday I will purchase any chicken that I am going to need for the Mon, Tues and Wednesday of the following week. On the Sunday I will prepare the right amount of meals that I will need to eat alongside my supplements to reach my protein target. Once cooked and I have left them to cool I will simply leave them in the fridge at a nice cool temperature. I personally wouldn't advise leaving them in the fridge for any longer than a couple of days but certainly within this period they are fine. Tuesday evening just before I am about to fun out on the Wednesday I will buy and cook for Thurs, Fri and Sat! How easy is that? Just 2 or 3 times cooking throughout the week and all meals are prepared! *Remember to use the packaging or an online search to find out the protein content of items and how close they take you towards your daily protein target.*

Protein before Bed?

One question I am regularly asked is what is the best time to STOP eating in the evening? Or is there a certain time that I am allowed to eat until? Although it's a very good question; there are a couple of responses which I swear by. OK, the first explanation is that it is certainly not the best option to eat a heavy meal or excessive carbohydrates just before bed; for the obvious reason that over the next couple of hours you will be using up less energy and therefore many of the calories are likely to store in the wrong places! However, if you remember in the section explaining the importance of breakfast I mentioned that whilst we sleep our body is rebuilding itself. Taking this into consideration; it is also important that we give our body a little bit of assistance through protein. Having a clean source of protein not too long before going to bed can limit muscle breakdown and also assist the body in its natural restoration while you sleep. So, my answer in short; If it's protein you are eating in the late evening this could actually assist with your goals. However, if it's a heavy source of calories and carbs I would definitely resist eating this.

Is it ok to have a cheat day?

Again, this is a topic that has so many science backed explanations with opposing views that it simply caused me to become a little confused. However, I am happy to share with you exactly what I have discovered through first-hand experience. I have personally noticed that when you follow a nice clean plan of nutrition day to day your results can sometimes come to a little plateaux. However, when providing my body with a "shock" and cheat meal every now and again, the high amount of sugars and carbohydrates almost cause the body to put up a defensive shield, your metabolism to work a little harder and therefore your body fat to decrease over the next couple of days when you are back to your clean nutrition plan. Now of course, a cheat day or cheat meals should not be integrated too frequently and you should not let one day feed into the next through bad disciplines and habits. I have always said that if you take one day of each week to indulge, then in a 30 day month that is just 4 days that weren't so great! Surely 4 is better than 30? And this also provides you with a nice pat on the back for your week consistency between cheat days.

Is there a specific time to have a post workout shake?

After working out it is very important that you are getting a blend of easily digestible proteins along with carbohydrates within 30 minutes of completing your training session. Something that is also very important to state here is that if you are training in the gym and you have a great burst of training for 10-15 minutes and then decide to stop for 10 minutes to speak with friends… And the cycle continues; this isn't the best method. This is because in my opinion your 30 minute window has already started once your muscles have gone a little cold during the 10 minute chat with your friends. My philosophy has always been to enter the gym and once I begin my 30-40 minute workout I do not stop working until I have finished my workout. And then within 30 minutes of me finishing my workout I must get a post workout recovery shake or good nutrition into my body. The reason I recommend post workout recovery shakes is because they are designed to enter your system quickly and simply speeds up the process of repairing and rebuilding the muscles.

How long should I train for to build bigger/more lean muscles?

During my training years I have been fortunate enough to meet so many people with different training goals and physique types. But I can honestly say that one gentleman in particular told me something that completely changed my life forever. He taught me that when aiming to develop a more fuller muscle or when building lean muscle mass; it is important that you simply quickly and efficiently damage the muscle through exercise and then get straight onto consuming the nutrition required to build that muscle. The reason this has been so important to me is because when I first met this particular individual I was spending at least 1-1 ½ hours in the gym working a muscle group per gym session. The first session I was fortunate enough to train with this gentleman was a session working arms, particularly biceps. As I walked into the gym, each piece of equipment was already set up and we went on to train 3 sets of 4 or 5 different exercises with minimum breaks between each set all within 10-15 minutes. 10-15 minutes? Yes you heard me correctly. And I understand that the bicep is one of the smaller muscles in our body, but these sessions continued throughout each muscle group spending no longer than 30-35 minutes on even some of the largest muscle groups within the body. During this particular period of time and into the present day I have never been able to gain lean muscle so quickly. This method combined with the right nutrition, could have me competition ready; far quicker than many of the time wasting regimes I have come across over the years. Let's think about this for just one moment. Each time we damage our muscles through weight training in particular, our muscles then require the correct nutrition and rest to rebuild. If you can damage the muscles as quickly and effectively as possible, this then offers more time for recovery and nutrition.

My Advice to guys and girls wanting to "bulk"

I want to touch on this topic very quickly because this is something that is very close to me. I am fortunate to have assisted so many guys and girls gain weight. Bulking in particular is of course about increasing calorie consumption. Right? But does that simply mean that we can fill our bodies with pretty much any type of calorie and call it "bulking"... Well if it's just gaining body fat in all of the wrong places including your stomach and face, then that's ok. But surely the actual aim of a "bulk" is to still have a nice handsome/pretty face but have some additional weight in the right places. When I speak to people who are wanting to go through this process. First of all I discuss that a "calorie" is not simply a "calorie" for example 1 calorie of chocolate is not the same as 1 calorie of broccoli and both will react completely different in the body. Next, I use an electronic scale and workout their Basal Metabolic Rate or BMR. This is the amount of calories that a person naturally burns each day due to the rate of their metabolism and muscle mass (The more muscle, the more calories they burn at rest). I then aim to increase their caloric intake by a minimum of 500kcal more than their BMR, this will ensure that they are having the correct amount of calories to put them on the right track. The next step is to set a step by step plan for these calories making sure that the calories they will be eating are also nutritious, there is nothing worse for somebody who wants to gain weight than simply eating empty calories which contain little or no nutritional value. For example, instead of them opting for a packet of crisps simply to get more calories into their system, why not a bowl of porridge oats? Instead of a fast food burger, why not a wholemeal grilled chicken wrap? Believe me, if a person can increase their calorie intake through sources of better nutrition they will see their overall weight increasing faster than ever before. Once their nutrition is set and I have made sure that they are also reaching their daily protein target and eating regularly; it's time to take a look at their training. Although the training is just 20% of their overall result, it is extremely important that the individual does not undo all of the hard work by simply spending too long in the gym, meaning that they expend too many calories and therefore have not consumed enough calories for that particular day. I advise my clients with the advice of "In and Out". Choose the muscle group that you would like to work, Carry out 3-4 sets on a heavier weight than you would normally choose (you should fail on no more than 6-8 reps). Put the weights back and then simply leave the gym! Simple right? It sounds simple, but you would be surprised if I told you how many times that I have come across people in gym's all around the world who spend hours in the gym burning calories with an attempt to "bulk" or "gain weight". It's important that you still remain fit and healthy and one way to do this whilst on your mission to gain weight is to go for a moderate stroll. By moderate, I mean not too fast at all, remember that the aim here is not to burn too many calories but simply to keep yourself, fit and mobile and to work the Cardio Vascular System at the same time.

If it's not in the cupboard, you won't eat it!

This is a topic that is very close to my heart. Just four months prior to writing this guide; I found myself in a position with a client who was relatively young. This particular individual was not yet old enough to do their own food shopping or even have the finances to do so. At the time of their visit; the young individual was quite heavily overweight and due to an underlying condition had been periodically told that if his habits did not change he would not have much time left to live. Upon hearing this I was surprised that any guardian would allow somebody who is their responsibility to get themselves into such a bad way. This brings me onto the topic of this section "If it's not in the cupboard, you can't eat it". When I asked the guardians of this particular individual exactly how the individual's food habits were, they explained that the individual would "sneak into the cupboards and snack on whatever they found". Imagine if there was nothing to be found? The point I am trying to make here; is if you are ready to get into the best shape of your life, you are going to have to make some sacrifices and decisions. The first would be to sit down with your family members or people you may live with; explain that you are going to be consistent with your new healthy lifestyle and invite them to join you on this new quest! Of course, this is not going to go down "a treat" (excuse the pun) with everyone as not everybody is ready to make that change at this moment in time (although prevention is better than cure). If this is the case; this is still a great opportunity to ask whether they could maybe hide some of the snacks that you may be tempted to cheat with. This doesn't need to become an Easter hunt! I simply mean rather than them being at the forefront of the kitchen cupboard each time you decide to open it; maybe they can keep their sugary snacks in a special draw that you don't need to open every day! I would also like to add at this point that if you are somebody who uses the "cheat day" technique in this guide; that you do not buy the treats in advance. For example. If cheat day comes around on a particular day of the week, then simply go out on the cheat day and purchase your items for that day. It is quite common that people will do so well on their nutrition plan and then suddenly when they finally think they have more self-control they will start buying their cheat day snacks in advance and promising not to touch them until the correct day. It's pretty obvious that it only takes a person to stub their toe on their way out of bed, or hear a little bit of "bad news" and before they know it they are eating their cheat day snacks on the wrong day! This requires real discipline and to be on the safe side I would suggest keeping your cupboards nice and clean (not literally) with food sources that fit into your "Motivator Meal Plan"

Does Everything Need to be Organic?

There is a huge myth in the present day that in order for food to become healthier and have the perfect physique. We must spend huge amounts of money on sourcing freshly grown, organic foods. Although this is true, that the food sources of today have far less nutritional content than in previous decades. I find that integrating meal replacements, supplements and wholefood sources into my diet not only contains far more micro nutrients (Vitamins and Minerals) but I also save money and time on the sourcing and preparation of my meals. The meats and fish used in my daily diet are not necessarily corn fed or organic, however I do believe that it is important that the meats purchased are of a good, fresh quality and have not been heavily treated or packaged for extended periods of time. I find that Ocean caught fish is a great lean source of protein and building a strong relationship with your local fish monger is never a bad idea!

How do I get a bigger bottom or behind? (One for the ladies)

We've arrived at the question that is at the tip of so many females tongues! How can I get a bigger bottom? Or larger glutes! It's important not to forget that the glutes are also a muscle. And how do we increase any muscle size in the body? We damage the muscle and then repair with the right amounts of protein and rest! There you have it! In order to get larger glutes and a more round behind I would firstly suggest researching and finding 4-5 effective glute exercises. Some great variations of these exercises can now be found online. These include both home workouts and gym workouts (Don't worry a gym is not necessarily required). Once you have planned the exercises that you would like to include in your session. Choose 2 days per week that you can spend 25-30 minutes carrying out these particular exercises. Now, there are a couple of nutrition aspects that are ital. to building this area. Firstly, it's absolutely imperative that after each session you complete; you have a post workout protein based shake or get the correct nutrition into your body within the 30 minute window. Believe me, this does not mean you are going to turn into a female body builder over night! Only a very tiny percentage of females carry the correct hormones to really build heavy muscle mass like a body builder. By simply increasing your protein; you will find that your physique actually becomes much slimmer (reduced body fat) along with an increase of tone. And of course the final piece to this section is to understand your protein target (muscle mass in pounds – The total amount of lbs of muscle is what you will need to consume daily in grams of protein) and make sure you are reaching this target as frequently as you can. After all this muscle cannot grow without the correct nutrition.

Is it ok for me to snack on fruit?

One of the things I am frequently asked is whether it is ok to snack on fruit throughout the day in order to reduce body fat. After all it is healthy right? The best way for me to describe this is for me to introduce you to my two friends once again. Friend number one has decided that he would like to become super healthy, one morning he wakes up and for the next couple of months decides that he is going to eat more fruit than ever before, he has a real thing for bananas and therefore starts having them between meals as a healthy snack. Meanwhile friend number 2 has also made a similar decision, however rather than snacking on fruits throughout the day; he decides to calculate his protein target using the method explained previously in the "protein" section of this guide; and then go about eating protein snacks between meals such as almond nuts or diced chicken breasts to reach his protein target. Within the first week or so there is no real difference between the results of friend number 1 and friend number 2. Friend number 1 has of course added extra vitamins and minerals to their overall diet through snacking on fruit and feels good. Friend number 2 has found their key vitamins and minerals in their meals but still has a focus on protein snacks between meals. After just a couple of weeks it now becomes more clear that whilst friend number 1 feels good he still weighs pretty much the same amount of weight and in fact his body fat has increased. Whereas by this point; friend number two has now started to reduce his body fat percentage, he is losing inches, looking fantastic. But of course because muscle weighs heavier than fat his overall weight may have even increased slightly. Result! Result? You ask? Why is that a result? When friend number 2 has gained weight? Well of course, this is the importance of body composition and understanding that the overall composition of your body is far more important than your weight alone on the scales.

Top Tip: Notice here that simply consuming more fruit to assist with a "diet" to lose body fat really isn't going to work. The increased amount of sugars simply that are not being used; simply start to create more body fat over time. And of course not achieving your protein target due to having fruit snacks instead of a protein source will also lead to losing your lean muscle mass. It's important to say at this point that I am by no means saying that an individual wanting to reduce body fat should not eat fruit. Fruit is a fantastic source of some of the most important vitamins, minerals and fibres. However, I just wanted to point out that there is simply more to it that just having a bit more fruit and believing you are "healthy" and on your way to your perfect body.

Let's take for example a gentleman who weighs 14st with 35% body fat and a gentleman who weighs 14st 8% body fat. One of which will categorically be over fat and the other under fat! Let's face it, have you ever heard a lady walk into a dress shop and ask for a 10 stone dress? Weight alone really doesn't prove anything, and this is where so many people become confused. Can you imagine the individual who decides to not eat much at all to lose weight, of course they are not reaching their protein target and therefore losing muscle mass each day. Remember muscle mass is the key driver to our metabolism and therefore muscle lost results in a body that is operating far less efficiently. Week on week this person continues to lose a couple of pounds in "weight" and feels fantastic, her friends and peers comment and congratulate her so therefore she continues to lose "weight" week by week. Once she has lost the desired amount of weight, she begins to break out of the consistency of her previous habit and starts to eat more freely again. But of course by this point, their metabolism is so slow and muscle mass is so low that there isn't much of an engine to burn through the calories coming into the body. What's the result? It's pretty obvious that this individual now gains back all of the weight that they have lost because they have not lost weight correctly. And this is what is known as a "yo-yo" dieter! Dieting and losing all of your muscle mass is certainly not the best practise to follow.

Consistency is Key

In summary I would like to share with you that my consistency and action have always been and will continue to be the most important aspects of my plan. It's a known fact that many people will simply read this guide, take the information on board and then find that applying the information just doesn't happen. I would like to ask that YOU yes YOU make the decision today to take those steps in the right direction, follow the ideas shared in this guide and begin to change your life TODAY!

I sincerely hope that this guide has helped you along your quest to be in the best shape of your life and can be used as a blueprint throughout your future! All the best! And enjoy your NEW BODY!

Kurt Motivator

"Don't lose your consistency, all it takes for your perfect physique

Is a little determination and consistency" – Kurt Motivator

"Being average is boring, aim to do something different to the average crowd" – Kurt Motivator

"Your thoughts and actions today,

are beginning to form your tomorrow" – Kurt Motivator

"Don't worry where you start out,

Focus on where you are going to finish" – Kurt Motivator

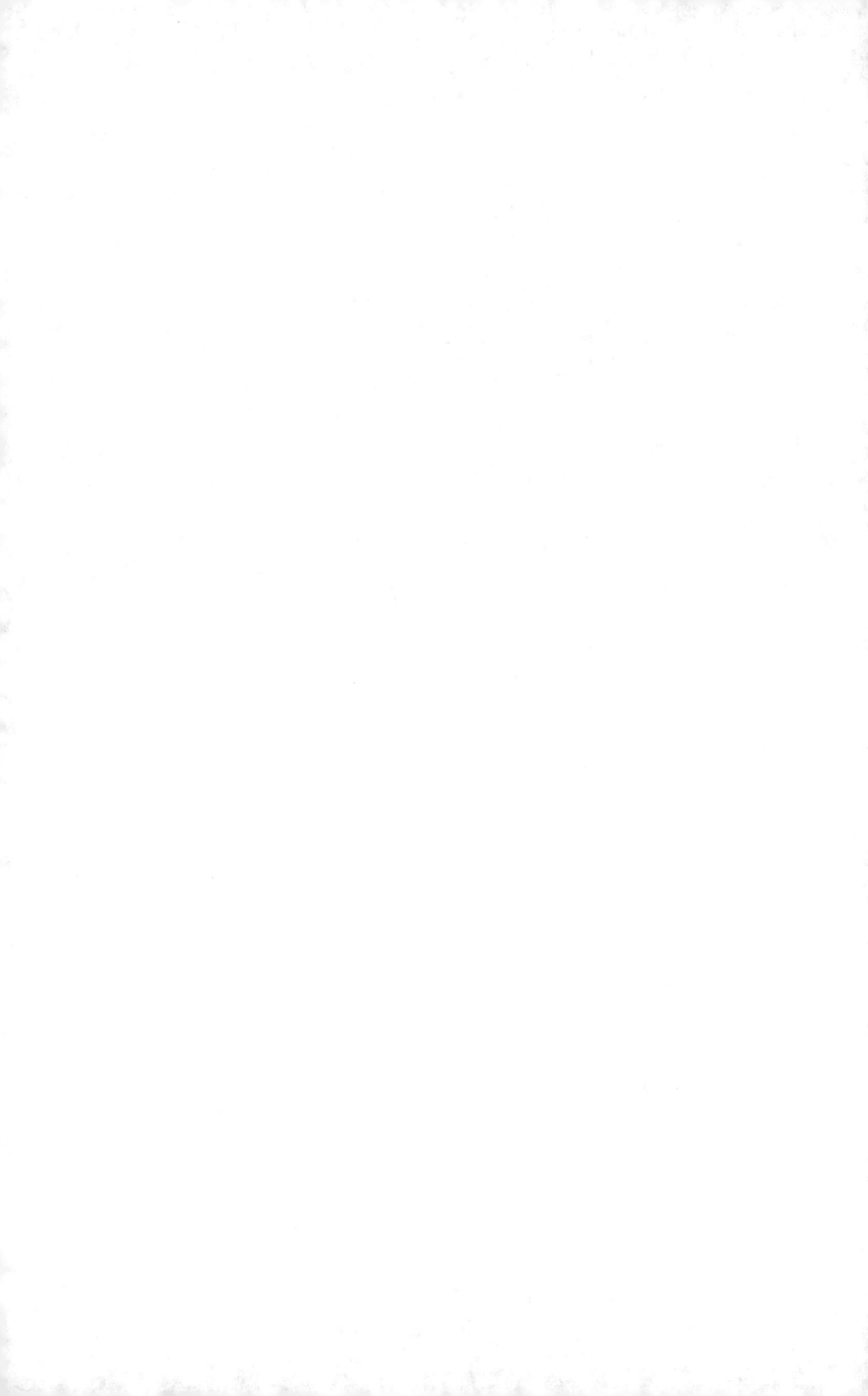

www.ingramcontent.com/pod-product-compliance
Lightning Source LLC
Chambersburg PA
CBHW072017280526
45788CB00005B/2075